AIF
COC
FOR
BEGINNERS
2021

CONTENTS

CONTENTS

CONTENTS

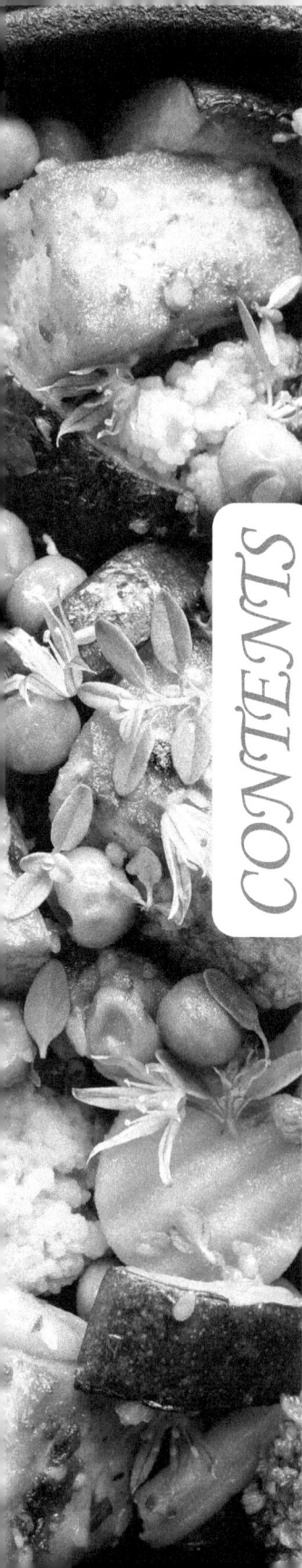

CONTENTS

Oregano and Sesame Sticks

Shopping List

- Agaragar in water

- Breadcrumbs

- Sesame

- Oregano

Instructions

Mix the agaragar together with the breadcrumbs until a dough is obtained. Form the sticks. Pass through a mix ture of oregano and sesame previously made. Place the sticks in the mold of the Air Fryer. Fry at 320 F for 8 15 minutes. Serve up

Crispy Bread with Guacamole

Shopping List

- 4 slices of bread

- Guacamole

- Anchovies in oil

Instructions

Cut the slices of bread into 3 strips. Coat with anchovy oil and add to the Air Fryer mold. Fry at 360 F for 10 minutes. Serve up the bread, on top of the guacamole and on top of it, the anchovies.

Vegetable Rolls

Shopping List

- Pack of rolls spring

- ½ cabbage cut into thin strips

- 2 large grated carrots

- Soy sauce

- Salt to taste

- Toasted sesame seeds

- Olive oil

- Creamy vegan cheese

Instructions

In a pan with a little oil, fry the vegetables over high heat. Add the soy sauce and salt. Leave the crispy vegetables. Remove from heat and let cool. Add the roasted sesame seeds. In a bowl mix the cream cheese with olive oil. Place the spring roll wrappers on the board and brush the sides with water. Add the sautéed on the wrap, fold the sides and roll up. Place in the mold of the Air Fryer previously varnished with olive oil, with the fold underneath. To varnish with the mixture of cheese and oil. Fry at 400 F for 5 10 minutes. Serve up with sweet and sour sauce.

Classic Pasties

Shopping List

- Salt

- ½ glass of sunflower oil

- Three cups of wheat flour

- ½ glass of water

Instructions

Boil the water off the heat and add the oil with the three cups of wheat flour, little by little. Stir with a wooden spoon, taking care that the lumps disappear and until it is impossible to continue stirring the dough. Let it cool and dump it in the meson. Knead with little hands until it does not stick from your hands. Cover with film and let stand for 1 hour. Serve up in 6 and stretch with the help of a rolling pin to a thickness of ½cm. Cut in a circle and fill. Rinse the edges with water and close. Add them to the Air Fryer programmed at 360 F for 8 12 minutes. Serve up hot with coffee.

Soy Patty

Shopping List

- 500gr wheat flour

- 1 can of soy meat

- Agaragar prepared in water

- 1 teaspoon salt

- 1 tablespoon Olive oil

- 1 cup of water

Instructions

Heat the water with the oil until warm. Place the flour, salt, and agar in a bowl. Add the water with oil. Knead until you get a bun. Reserve up with plastic film for a ½ hour. Season the soy meat to taste and Reserve up. Stretch the dough and fill the patty. Close them and seal them. Place in the Air Fryer and fry at 360 F for 7 minutes. Serve up hot.

Endives with Honey Vinaigrette

Shopping List

- 2 endives in half

- 2 kinds of garlic, mashed

- 2 apples in sheets

- Olive oil

- Salt and pepper

- Balsamic vinegar

- Honey

Instructions

Place the endives in the mold of the Air Fryer. Bathe with garlic oil and salt. Schedule at 360 F for 20 25 minutes. Meanwhile, mix honey and vinegar in equal parts with oil. Serve up the endives garnishing with apple and on top the honey vinaigrette.

Caesar Vegan Salad

Shopping List

- 1 Washed romaine lettuce

- Soy sauce

- Water

- Thyme

- Paprika

- Garlic powder

- Onion powder

- Pepper

- Tofu cut into cubes

- 250ml Vegan Caesar sauce

- Parmesan cheese

Instructions

Add the tofu in the Air Fryer programmed at 360 F for 15 minutes. Half cooked, turn to brown all sides. Meanwhile, mix the soy sauce, water, and spices. Add the tofu and stir to impregnate. Sauté in a pan for 5 minutes over high heat and set aside. Place the chopped lettuce, add the tofu, parmesan, and stir. Serve up as a companion or with croquettes.

Mediterranean Vegetables

Shopping List

- 50g of cherry tomatoes

- 1 large cut zucchini

- 1 green pepper cut

- 1 large parsnip cut

- 1 medium carrot cut

- 1 teaspoon mixed herbs

- 2 tablespoons of honey

- 1 tablespoon mustard

- 2 tablespoons of mashed garlic

- Olive oil

- Salt and pepper

Instructions

In the mold of the Air Fryer, place the zucchini, green pepper, parsnip, carrot and whole cherry tomatoes. Add a little olive oil and stir. Fry at 360 F for 15 minutes. Meanwhile in a bowl mix the herbs, mustard, honey, garlic and a drizzle of olive oil. When you finish the veg etables, remove and place in the bowl and mix well. Re turn the mixture to the Air Fryer and fry at 400 F for 5 8 minutes. Serve up.

Fried Asparagus with Pepper

Shopping List

- ½ bunch of asparagus

- Olive oil

- Salt and pepper

Instructions

Cut 5 cm from the base of the asparagus. Place them in the mold of the Air Fryer. Lightly spray with oil and sprinkle with salt and pepper. Fry at 400 F for 8 10 minutes. Serve up hot

Sweet N 'Chips

Shopping List

- Sweet potato in cubes

- Cornmeal

- Olive oil

- Paprika

- Salt and pepper

- Garlic and onion powder

Instructions

Cook the sweet potatoes in a pot of water with salt. When softening, process with the rest of the Shopping Listexcept the flour. If there is no liquid, use the cooking water. Place the mixture in a bowl and add flour to form a firm dough. On paper film painted with oil, place the dough and cover with more film. Stretch with a roller until thin. Cut the wafers with a cup. Sprinkle with more garlic and onion. Take the Air Fryer programmed at 360 F for 4 8 minutes. Let cool and Serve up alone or with sauce.

Filled Tomatoes

Shopping List

- 6 washed tomatoes

- 2 onions in cubes

- 200g vegetarian cheese sliced

- Parsley finely cut

- Olive oil

- Salt and pepper

Instructions

Cut the lid of the tomatoes and extract the pulp. Sauté the onions. Add tomato, salt, and pepper. Mix well and let cool. Add the cheese and fill the tomatoes. Place the lid, varnish them with olive oil and take them to the mold of the Air Fryer programmed at 360 F for 30 minutes. Serve up hot.

Natural Artichokes

Shopping List

- Artichokes

- Olive oil

- Salt and pepper

Instructions

Remove the first layers of the artichoke. Cut the tip and stem. Tap lightly above to open, season and varnish with oil. Take them to the Air Fryer programmed at 360 F for 12 15 minutes. Thoroughly varnish the center with oil and program again for another 10 minutes. Remove the drier leaves and Serve up hot.

Potatoes with Mushrooms

Shopping List

- 500g fine skin potatoes

- ½ lemon juice

- Thyme

- Olive oil

- 200g of mushrooms in half

- Salt and pepper

- Breadcrumbs.

Instructions

Cut the potatoes into medium pieces and place them in the mold of the Air Fryer. Bathe with lemon, thyme, and oil. Incorporate the mushrooms and mix everything. Season and program it at 360 F for 10 15 minutes. Mix and sprinkle with bread. Program it again for 25 30 minutes. Serve up hot.

Salad Of Rice and Avocados

Shopping List

- 2 avocados in slices

- 1 cup of rice

- 1 can of drained peas

- 2 spring onions julienne

- 1 cucumber

- 1 tablet of chicken broth

- 1 carrot in small cubes

- Stuffed Olives

- Olive oil

- Lemon juice

- Salt, pepper, and water

Instructions

In the mold of the Air Fryer add the rice, a little oil, and salt. Mix and program it at 360 F for 10 15 minutes. Let cool. Mix pepper, oil, lemon juice and the shredded pill. Mix all the Shopping Listwith the rice and add the previous vinaigrette. Serve up fresh

Baklava

Shopping List

- 1 sheet of puff pastry

- 300g Mani

- Melted butter

- Honey

- Water

- Lemon juice

- sugar

- Cinnamon

Instructions

Process the peanut until obtaining a thick paste and Reserve up. Cut the puff pastry in 8 and stretch until it is millimeters thick. To varnish one of the sheets with but ter, to sprinkle with peanuts and to bathe with honey. Place another sheet on top and repeat until the materials are exhausted. Cut into small squares and take the Air Fryer programmed at 360 F for 30 40 minutes. Let stand 15 minutes. Meanwhile, place in a pot water, sugar, lemon juice, cinnamon and stir until boiling and thickening. Let the previously made dough rest and bathe. Rest for 1 hour and Serve up with coffee or tea.

Flavored Tomatoes

Shopping List

- 8 tomatoes sliced in 2

- Grated cheese

- Garlic and parsley

- Salt and pepper

- Olive oil

Instructions

In a bowl mix everything to taste except tomatoes. Place the tomatoes in the mold of the Air Fryer with the skin facing down and bathe with the previous mixture. Process it at 360 Ffor 10 15 minutes. Serve up as an entree or garnish for meats.

Vegetables with Marinated Feta

Shopping List

- 800g Cauliflower in florets

- 400g Pumpkin in canes

- Ground cumin

- Paprika

- 1 Lemon

- 200g Feta cheese in cubes

- 1 garlic, mashed

- 5g laminated and dried chili pepper

- Rosemary

- Olive oil

- Salt and pepper

- 15ml of soy sauce

Instructions

Place cauliflower and squash in the mold of the Air Fryer adding cumin, paprika, salt, lemon juice, soy sauce and olive oil. Stir well and set at 360 F for 25 30 minutes. Meanwhile, toast garlic, chili, rose mary and re moves from heat, let cool and add cheese. Serve up the vegetables with cheese and marinate on top.

Pinch Skewers

Shopping List

- 1 Fresh temples

- 300g Tofu in cubes

- Basil leaves

- Bamboo sticks for skewers

- Parisian spoon

- Wheat flour with water

Instructions

To bathe the tofu pieces the mixture of flour and to take them to the Air Fryer programmed to 360 F by 5 10 minutes. Meanwhile, remove the seeds from the pin and cut balls with the Parisian spoon. Prepare the skewers alternating tofu, pin and basil leaves. Serve up fresh

Potatoes with Broccoli

Shopping List

- 300g of sliced potato

- 300g of shelled broccoli

- 1 tablet of chicken broth

- Olive oil

- Breadcrumbs

- Salt and pepper

Instructions

In a pan of boiling water add the broccoli for 1 minute. To bathe the potatoes with oil, the crumbled tablet, salt, pepper and to mix. In the mold of the previously greased Air Fryer, add a layer of potatoes, then cover with broccoli and finish with potatoes. Schedule at 360 F for 20 25 minutes. Serve up hot

Lemon Artichokes

Shopping List

- 6 artichokes

- Olive oil

- 1 tablet of chicken broth

- Parsley finely cut

- Pepper

- Juice and leftovers of 1 lemon

Instructions

Remove the first layers of the artichoke and varnish with lemon. Grease the mold of the Air Fryer and place the artichokes. Bathe with oil, lemon juice, and the shred ded pill. Schedule at 360 F for 12 18 minutes. Serve up hot

VEGETARIAN RECIPES

Surprises of Taro with White Cheese

Shopping List

- 1/2 of taro

- 2 Cloves of garlic

- Chopped parsley

- Shredded white cheese

- Chopped sweet peppers

- 1 Whole eggs

- Salt

Instructions

Grate the taros and place them in a glass bowl. Mix with the other Shopping Listexcept for the grated cheese. Let it rest in the refrigerator with plastic wrap, for ½ hour. Form balls and introduce enough grated cheese inside. Seal and bring to the Air Fryer for 35 minutes at 320 F. Check the cooking and flip. Fry for 35 more minutes. Serve up very hot, tiny as snacks and large as company ions.

Morning Corn with Cheese

Shopping List

- 1 ½ Cup of Tender Corn

- 250g of chopped cheese

- 2 onions.

- 6 Eggs

- Salt.

- Pepper.

- Grated cheese.

Instructions

Beat the eggs with salt and pepper. Add the cheese, onion, and corn and mix well. Grease the mold of the fryer and pour the tortilla. Set the fryer for 1015 at 360 F per minute. Serve up with butter and grated cheese. Garnish with corn and parsley.

Lentil Tortilla with Cheese

Shopping List

- Cooked lentils.

- Cheese.

- Margarine.

- Salt.

- Water

Instructions

Take the lentil and grind to the processor. Place in a bowl and add the rest of the Shopping List. Grease the mold of the fryer and place the mixture with the help of a large spoon. Put in the Air Fryer for 10 15 minutes at a temperature of 320 F. Flip to fry on the other side. They a Reserved up with butter and cheese.

Rolled Courgettes with Oregano

Shopping List

- 3 Courgettes

- 220g of creamy goat cheese.

- Salt

- Whole black pepper.

- 150g of whole Parmesan cheese.

- Olive oil.

Instructions

Wash and cut zucchini along. Coat with olive oil and pour into the Air Fryer for 4 minutes at 360 F. Remove the slices of courgettes from the fryer and let cool. Apart crush the goat cheese. Grind the pepper. Mix the cheese with salt and pepper. Place this Instructionson the zuc chini slices and roll up. Fix with chopsticks. Place in molds and place goat cheese on top. Bring back to the Air Fryer for 812 minutes at 360 F. When ready, sprinkle parmesan cheese on top and Se

Serrve up with tomato sauce with oregano.

Cheese Fingers

Shopping List

- 500 g hard cheese cut into 6x1 strips

- 500 grams of breadcrumbs

- Parmesan

- Parsley finely chopped

- 1 tablespoon garlic powder

Instructions

Mix cheese, bread, parsley and garlic powder in a bowl. Go through the breaded each cheese finger. Place them in the Air Fryer without over coating them. Fry at 360 F for 4 to 8 minutes. Serve up hot accompanied by the sauce of preference.

Spanish omelet with Zucchini

Shopping List

- ½ cup of olive oil

- ½ sliced zucchini

- Pepper

- 1 Large onion

- 4 eggs

- Salt.

- Pepper.

- 2 tomatoes

- 2 green onions,

Instructions

Wash the tomatoes and take out the seed. Chop into large pieces. Chop the onions and mix with the zucchini; salt and pepper scramble the eggs with salt and pepper. Place a little olive oil in the mold of the Air Fryer and pour the zucchini and onion. Fry for 1 minute. Move and add the Instructionsof the eggs. Stir well and bring to fry again for 10 15 minutes at 320 F. Serve up hot, with toasted bread or to taste.

Eggplant and Cheese Croquettes

Shopping List

- 500 g of eggplant

- 100 g of semihard vegan cheese

- 200 ml of vegetable milk

- 20 grams of flour

- 1 onion

- Nutmeg

- Black pepper

- Oregano

- Salt

- 2 eggs

- Flour or Breadcrumbs

- Olive oil

Instructions

Roast the eggplants on the grill, on the stove or in the oven; as you prefer Let cool a little, peel and crush. Reserve up. Add flour, grated cheese, and oregano. Mix well and take it to the refrigerator until the dough is cold. Make small balls.

Spinach and Ricotta Cheese Crepes

Shopping List

- 1 cup of wheat flour

- 1 ½ cups of milk

- Olive oil

- ½ teaspoon baking powder

- 1 kilo of spinach

- 2 tablespoons of water

- 2 tablespoons finely chopped scallion

- 1 cup ricotta cheese

- ¼ cup of Parmesan cheese

- Salt and pepper to taste

Instructions

In the blender process the flour, milk, a little oil and the baking powder. Meanwhile, in boiling water dip the spinach. Take them out and dry them. Cut them finely

and mix with green onions, cheese, nutmeg, salt, and pepper. Reserve up. In the mold of the Air Fryer painted with olive oil, place the mixture forming crepes. Fry at 300 F for 6 to 10 minutes. Place the filling in the crepes and another crepe on top. Sprinkle with Parmesan cheese and fry at 280 F for 5 minutes. Serve up hot

Banana Tempura

Shopping List

- 6 bananas

- 1 cup of wheat flour

- 2 egg yolks

- 3/4 cups of water

- 1 tbsp Of sugar

- Bamboo sticks

- Strawberry syrup

Instructions

Cut the bananas in half. In a bowl add flour, yolks, water, and sugar. Mix. Pass the bananas through the mixture and place them in the Air Fryer. Fry at 360 F for 5 minutes. Serve up on a plate accompanied by strawberry syrup.

Sweet Corn Pancake

Shopping List

- Tender corn.

- 1 Cup of cornmeal.

- 1 Cup of Milk

- 1 Cup of grated cheese.

- 1 teaspoon salt.

- 1 teaspoon of Sugar

- Butter.

Instructions

Place the tender corn in the processor. In a bowl mix all the Shopping Listvery well. The dough must be manageable. Make the disc shaped pancakes and take them to the Air Fryer for 1015 minutes at 360 F. Serve up and spread with butter and accompany it with a soft cheese, to taste.

Banana Rolls

Shopping List

- 3 ripe bananas.

- Optional English sauce

- 1 egg

- Wheat flour.

- 1 onion

- 200g of soy meat

- Olives

- Sweet pepper

- Garlic

- Dressing

Instructions

Hydrate the meat for 10 minutes. Drain very well. Peel and chop the bananas in half in two slices each. To part, marinate the meat and fry with the garlic. Add the other minced Shopping Listto the meat. Form circles with the slices and fix it with the chopsticks. Fill with the soy meat; let it rest a little so that the liquid comes out. Seal with egg and a little wheat flour. Place in the fryer for 8 15 minutes at 320 F. Watch the cooking, turn to cook evenly.

Fried Polenta

Shopping List

- 100g of precooked cornmeal

- ½ L of water

- 25gr of butter

- Salt to taste

- Oil

Instructions

Put the water in a pot, when boiling; pour the cornmeal in the form of rain. Mix vigorously with a wooden spoon. Lower the heat to a minimum and continue beating for 6 to 8 minutes, without stopping. Add salt and butter, continue beating.

Drop the polenta from the fire and pour it into a square tray and make sure the thickness is 1 centimeter. When the polenta has cooled, place it on the work surface and cut into sticks. Fry in Air Fryer for 1015 minutes at 360 F. This versatile Instructionsis served up to taste.

Have three dishes; One dish with flour, another with two beaten eggs and the third with Breadcrumbs. Go through each plate, one by one and in the order indicated the meatballs. Bring the Air Fryer for 1015 minutes at 360 F. It is ac companied with bread, rice, steamed potatoes or boiled cassava.

Banana Stew with Maple Honey

Shopping List

- 3 bananas

- 1/2 cup flour

- 1 egg yolks

- Water

- 1 tablespoon sugar

- Bamboo sticks

- Honey of maple

Instructions

Peel and chop the bananas in half. Mix the other Shopping Listvery well, so it becomes thick. Spread the chambers by the previous mixture and Fry in Air Fryer for 35 minutes at 320 F. Check cooking and flip. Fry for 35 minutes more. Serve up and bathe with maple honey and place a touch of cinnamon or taste.

Stuffed Corn Moons

Shopping List

- ½ cup of milk

- 4 Sweet young corns.

- Cornmeal.

- Striped white cheese.

- Salt.

- 1 teaspoon of sugar (optional)

Instructions

Place the corn in the processor and grind very well. Pour the ground corn into a bowl, add the milk, salt, grated cheese, and flour and knead very well. Form the dough discs and place cheese on them. Close and fry in Air Fryer for 815 minutes at 320 F.

Carbonara's Tortilla.

Shopping List

- 4 sliced potatoes

- 1 onion in julienne

- 100g Vegan Bacon

- 5 beaten eggs

- Grated cheese

- Nutmeg

- Salt

Instructions

Place the potatoes and onions in the Air Fryer at 320 F for 20 minutes. Meanwhile, in a pan, fry the bacon without oil until golden brown. Reserve. Let the potatoes cool. Beat the eggs vigorously. Add the potatoes, onion, bacon, cheese, and nutmeg. Mix well all the Shopping List. Add the tortillas to the Air Fryer and set at 360 F for 20 minutes.

Cassava Balloons with Cheese

Shopping List

- ½ kg of cassava.

- 1 cup of flour.

- 100g of cheese

- 1 egg.

- Salt.

- Pepper.

Instructions

Parboil yucca Grind with all the Shopping List. Place a piece of cheese in the center. Close and go through the beaten egg. Then go through wheat flour. Put it in Air Fryer for 68 minutes at 360 F. Flip.

Fried Corn

Shopping List

- 2 Cans of corn.

- 2 Eggs

- 1 chopped onion

- 3 garlic cloves.

- 2 table spoon of parsley.

- 2 table spoon of wheat flour.

- 1/2 Teaspoon of baking powder

- Salt

Instructions

Drain the corn very well. Separate a portion. Blend or process all the Shopping List. Add the whole grains that you had separated and mix very well. Grease the mold surface of the Air Fryer and fry for 810 minutes at 360 F. Check the cooking and turn to finish cooking.

Bean Roll

Shopping List

- 300 gr of beans

- 2 onions cut in julienne

- 1 zucchini cut into cubes

- 4 potatoes cut into cubes

- 8 eggs

- Olive oil

- Salt and pepper

- A little soy sauce Instructions

Instructions

In a pot of water, cook the beans with salt. Being tender drain and reserve up. Place the potatoes in the mold of the Air Fryer. Season and place oil threads, mix and fry at 360 F for 15 minutes. Add the zucchini and onion, mix and fry at 360 F for 10 minutes. Stir and place another 10 minutes. Pass the contents of the Air Fryer to a pan with the beans. Add soy sauce and salt and pepper. Sauté, crack the eggs and make the scramble. Serve up hot.

Weekend Sandwich

Shopping List

- 12 Sandwich bread

- 12 slices of turkey ham

- 6 slices of vegan cheese

- 1½ cups of grated yellow cheese

- 1 cup of milk cream

- 100 g of Butter

- Salt and pepper to taste

Instructions

First, spread a little butter on the bread slices. Place one of the loaves, two slices of ham, one of cheese and close. Place in the Air Fryer and fry at 300 F for 2 minutes. Meanwhile, in a bowl, mix the cheese, cream, salt, and pepper. Cover the sandwich with the mixture. Fry at 340 F for 4 minutes until golden brown. Serve up hot.

Adventure Overflowing Bread

Shopping List

- Homemade bread

- Milk and cinnamon

- Eggs

- Honey

- 4 tablespoons of Sugar

- 1 glass of water Instructions

Instructions

First, cut the slices of bread and Reserve up. Heat the milk with cinnamon. When boiling, remove from heat and set aside. Beat the eggs. Bathe the bread in the milk, then the egg and drain. Place the bread in the mold of the Air Fryer without stacking. Fry at 360 F for 10 minutes. Place the honey in a pot with water and sugar. When boiling remove from heat. Pass the bread through the honey and let cool. Serve up cold.

Provocative Ace mite of Corn

Shopping List

- 1½ cups of sweet corn

- 1 tablespoon Of Flour

- 1 tablespoon of baking powder

- 2 eggs

- 4 tablespoon of sugar

- ½ tsp of salt

- Butter

Instructions

In the blender process the corn, eggs, flour, sugar, baking powder, and salt. Glaze the mold of the Air Fryer with melted butter. Pour a little of the mixture making small cakes. Fry at 360 F for 4 7 minutes until crispy. Serve up with a sauce preferably or sprinkled with sugar.

Vegetable Cheesecake

Shopping List

- 4 wheat flour tortillas

- 1 cup of Cheddar cheese

- 1 cup sliced red pepper

- 1 cup of sliced zucchini

- 1 cup of drained canned beans

- 60g of Greek yogurt

- 1 teaspoon lime zest

- 1 tablespoon lime juice

- ¼ teaspoon cumin

- 2 tablespoons chopped coriander

- ½ cup of peak of rooster

- Olive oil

Instructions

Sprinkle grated cheese over half the cheesecake. Cover with a ¼ cup of red peppers, zucchini, and beans. Sprinkle with the rest of the cheese. Close the tortillas and sprinkle with olive oil, securing them with toothpicks. Carefully place the quesadillas in the Air Fryer and fry at 400 F for 5 minutes. Flip and fry for 5 more minutes. Meanwhile, in a bowl, mix the yogurt, the zest and the lime juice with the cumin. Serve up the quesadilla cut into pieces. Serve up with 2 tablespoons Pico de Gallo and a spoonful of yogurt cream.

Spinach Nugget

Shopping List

- 360g Spinach

- 200 ml Spinach water

- 70g Wheat flour

- 1 Finely cut onion

- 50ml milk

- 20g Butter

- 1 Clove of garlic, mashed

- Nutmeg

- Olive oil

- Pepper

- Salt

- 2 eggs beaten with salt

- Breadcrumbs

Instructions

In a pot of boiling water, add the spinach for 8 minutes. Drain and recover the water that drains. Cut finely. In a pan, add butter and oil. Sauté the onion 2 minutes. Add the garlic and sauté. Add the spinach, season and sauté 3 minutes. Integrate the flour and cook stirring for 3 minutes. Place the milk, water, salt and pepper and mix until you get a dough. Remove from heat and let cool. Shape the nuggets.

Pass through egg and Breadcrumbs Add to the Air Fryer.

Fry at 360 F for 5 to 8 minutes.

Serve up alone or with the preferred sauce.

Potato Cake

Shopping List

- 4 Sliced potatoes

- 300g Bacon

- 200g Sliced cheese

- Grated cheese

- 2 eggs

- Salt and pepper

- 200ml milk cream

- Olive oil

- 1 onion in julienne

Instructions

Mix the beaten eggs with the cream, season and Reserve up. Pepper the potatoes. Coat the mold of the Air Fryer with oil. Place a layer of potatoes, then onions, bacon, cheese and more potatoes. On top add a little of the egg mixture. Repeat until the Shopping Listare used up. In the last layer of potatoes, add the mixture and sprinkle with grated cheese. Cover with aluminum foil and put the Air Fryer at 360 F for 40 minutes. Missing 10 minutes, remove the foil and gratin. Serve up alone.

Tender Corn Pancake

Shopping List

- Sweet corn

- 1 Mug of corn flour.

- 1 Cup of Leche.de soy

- 1 Cup of Vegan grated cheese.

- 1 tsp of Sal.

- 1 Cake of Sugar

- Butter

Instructions

Place tender corn on the processor. In a bowl mix all the Shopping List very well. Must be the manageable dough. Make the disk shaped jackets and take them to the Air Fryer for 812 minutes at 360 F. Serve up and spread with butter and accompanied with a soft cheese, to taste.

Mamma Mía Potatoes

Shopping List

- ½ Kg of potatoes

- 2 Eggs

- 1/2 can of evaporated milk

- 1/2 cube of chicken

- ¼ cup of butter.

- ¼ of the creamy vegan cheese

Instructions

Peel and cut the potatoes in fine wheels. Make a smooth paste with the eggs, milk, cube, and butter. In the greased mold, layers of potatoes are placed alternately with cream and layers of cheese, making sure that the last layer is cream. Take the Air Fryer for 1527 minutes at 360 F, then check the cooking.

Rosemary Potatoes

Shopping List

- 24 Colombian potatoes

- 100g of butter

- 6 cloves of garlic mashed

- 3 branches of rosemary

- Sea salt

Instructions

Wash and dry the potatoes well. Place the butter with garlic and rosemary on the Air Fryer. Fry at 300 F for 1 minute. Add potatoes, salt and mix well. Cover with foil and fry at 340 F for 15 minutes. Then discover and fry for 5 more minutes. Serve up as a garnish for fish.

Pumpkin Buns with Cheese Surprise

Shopping List

- ½ kg of peeled pumpkin.

- ½ kg of annealed corn flour.

- Salt. Pepper to taste.

- White cheese grated.

- Pieces of cheese

- Ham Sticks.

- Wheat flour.

Instructions

Mix the Shopping Listwell. Form small balls. Open a hole in the center and introduce a piece of cheese and ham. Close, go through a beaten egg, then wheat flour. Place in the spectacular Air Fryer and fry for 812 minutes, at 360 F. It is Serve up with sauces, salads or melted cheese; according to taste.

Crunchy Nuts

Shopping List

- 4 Slices of bread
- 2 large eggs
- ¼ cup of milk
- 1 teaspoon vanilla
- ½ teaspoon ground cinnamon
- ¼ cup of brown sugar
- ⅔ cups of flax seed meal
- Bean Croquettes
- Shopping List
- 100g green beans
- 3 carrots cut into small cubes
- 300 ml thick béchamel
- Breadcrumbs
- Chickpea flour
- Water
- Virgin olive oil
- Salt

Instructions

First, place the beans and carrots in a pan and sauté. When softened add salt and mix with the thick béchamel. Let it stand for 2 hours until it hardens. Mix the flour with the water until you get a light cream. with the help of a spoon take portions of the béchamel mixture. Sprinkle in the flour mixture and bathe in Bread crumbs. Shape it into croquettes and place in the Air Fryer. Fry for 5 7 minutes until browned and removed. Serve up with salad.

Spicy Cheese Meatballs

Shopping List

- 600g Cheddar cheese in cubes

- 240g Clean Chilies

- 2 eggs beaten with salt

- Doritos

- Olive oil

Instructions

In a processor, add half of the Chilies and cheese until you have a paste. Cut the rest of the chilies finely and incorporate them into the dough. Knead until integrating all the chilies. Grind the Doritos to make a powder. Assemble the meatballs. Pass them by egg and Doritos. Brush them with olive oil and add them to the Air Fryer. Fry at 360 F for 5 to 8 minutes. Serve up with yogurt sauce, alone or with pink sauce

Malanga and Cheese Fritters.

Shopping List

- ½ Kg of grated malanga

- 4 cloves garlic, mashed

- 1/2 cup of cut parsley

- 200 g. of grated white cheese

- 1/2 Cup of chopped sweet peppers

- 2 Whole eggs

- Salt to taste

Instructions

Place the malanga grated in a large bowl. Process the garlic, chili, and parsley. Add to malanga. Add the beaten eggs and salt and pepper. Knead until compact. Cover with plastic wrap and Reserve up in the fridge. Once cold, shape the donuts and place them in the mold of the Air Fryer. Fry at 360 F for 8 to12 minutes. Serve up and accompany it with the sauce of preference.

Fried Snacks

Shopping List

- 4 Potatoes with skin on sticks

- 2 Eggs

- 1 Onion in small cubes

- Chilies to taste

- Barbecue sauce

- Ketchup

- Honey

- Wheat flour

Instructions

Add the onion in a bowl and add flour. Add the potatoes with salt to the mold of the Air Fryer, and program it at 360 F for 8 15 minutes. After 10 minutes add the onions and mix so that everything is crispy. In a pan fry the eggs and Chilies. Meanwhile, mix the BBQ sauce, ketchup, and honey. Serve up by placing the potatoes, over the eggs and chilies and a little of the sauce.

Olive oil

- 2 cups sliced strawberries

- 8 teaspoons maple syrup

- 1 teaspoon of sugar glass

Instructions

First, cut each slice of bread in 4 lengthwise. In a bowl, beat the eggs, milk, vanilla, cinnamon and 1 tablespoon of brown sugar. Aside, mix the flour and the remaining brown sugar. Dip the bread in the egg mixture and drain. Pass through the flour mixture and cover with olive oil. Place in the mold of the Air Fryer and fry at 360 F for 5 minutes. Flip and fry for 5 more minutes. Serve up with the strawberries accompany it with the maple syrup and sprinkling with icing sugar.

Venezuelan Arepas

Shopping List

- 160g corn flour

- 300ml water

- Salt

- Olive oil

- 100g turkey ham

- 100g sliced cheese

- Butter

Instructions

In a bowl mix the water and salt to taste. Stir and add the flour. Mix until a medium solids paste is obtained. Let stand 5 10 minutes. Knead a little and check the texture, if it is solid add a little more water. Form some balls the size of your hands. Go crushing little by little in a circular way with your hands to form a disc 1 cm thick. Place the arepas in the Air Fryer, and set at 360 F for 10 to 15 minutes. Half the time turns around. Serve up, open one of the sides with a knife. Add butter, cheese or another filling preferably. Accompany it with coffee or natural juice

White Tortilla

Shopping List

- 2 halfmoon courgettes

- 1 Eggplant in a half moon

- 1 Onion in feathers

- 5 beaten eggs

- Olive oil

- Soy sauce

Instructions

Sauté in a pan with oil, onion, zucchini, and eggplant. Add salt, soy sauce and sauté. Add to the Air Fryer mold and add the eggs with salt. Set at 320 F for 25 minutes. Serve up with sautéed vegetables.

Chip N' Sitos

Shopping List

- 2 potatoes in thin slices

- 2 eggs

- ½ julienne onion

- 1 package of bacon

- Olive oil

- Salt

Instructions

Wash the potatoes in abundant water. Drain and dry. Heat the oil in a pan and sauté the onions; Reserve up. Fry the egg with a pinch of salt and cover; Reserve up. In the Air Fryer place the potatoes at 360 F for 5 minutes until golden brown, and Reserve up. Add the bacon to the Air Fryer at 360 F for 5 10 minutes. Serve up placing the potatoes, on them the onion, more potatoes and especially the egg. Place the bacon on its side, dropping it.

Quick Zucchini's Tortilla

Shopping List

- 2 sliced zucchini

- 1 Onion in julienne

- 4 beaten eggs

- Salt

Instructions

Sauté the onion and zucchini in a pan. Add everything to the Air Fryer mold and program it at 320 F for 20 25 minutes. Serve up with bread and coffee or natural juice.

Garlic's Tortilla

Shopping List

- 1 onion in julienne

- 4 Potatoes in thin slices

- 4 kinds of garlic, mashed

- Parsley finely cut

- 4 Eggs

Instructions

Take and place the onions and potatoes in the Air Fryer at 360 F for 5 minutes. Mix the garlic, parsley, and eggs. Add the fried potatoes and onions. Mix and empty the mixture in a pan over low heat. Set and Serve up the tor tile. Accompany it bread or corn cakes.

Loroco's Arepas

Shopping List

- ½Kg Corn Flour

- 1L of water

- Salt

- 2 cups washed lorocos

- 500g of grated cheese

Instructions

Process the lorocos with the water in the blender. Place in a bowl and add salt to taste. Add the flour and cheese. Mix, knead and let stand for 5 minutes. Knead again and incorporate water if necessary. Form balls the size of your hands and crush them to form discs 1cm thick. Place them in the Air Fryer at 360 F for 10 15 minutes. Halfway through cooking. Serve up stuffed like a Venezuelan Arepa.

Basil Lasagna

Shopping List

- 1 Package of lasagna pasta

- 2 cups of milk

- 2 Tbs. of wheat flour

- 1 Grated onion

- 1 Pinch of nutmeg

- 2 Tbs. of butter

- 1 Cup of crushed basil

- 250 g. of cottage cheese with salt

- 100 g of grated parmesan

- Salt and pepper to taste

Instructions

In the blender add milk, flour, nutmeg, salt, a table spoon of butter and process. Place a pot with the rest of the butter and onion. Sweat it and add the blender mixture. Mix until thickening and Reserve up. Meanwhile, in a bowl add the ricotta cheese with salt and basil. Serve up. In boiling salted water cook the pasta, until it is al dente. In the mold of the Air Fryer assemble the lasagna. Place a little white sauce on the bottom, then the pasta and the ricotta filling, and so on. When finished cover with white sauce and sprinkle parmesan cheese. Cover with aluminum foil and fry at 360 F for 15 minutes. Remove the foil and fry again for 5 minutes until golden brown. Serve up hot

Tortilla's Dice

Shopping List

- Olive oil

- 300g onion in small cubes

- 1kg potato in small cubes

- Salt

- 10 beaten eggs

Instructions

In the mold of the Air Fryer place a little oil, and sauté the potatoes with the onions and a pinch of salt; at 360 F for 25 30 minutes, stirring periodically. Add the beaten eggs with a pinch of salt and stir. Schedule 15 to 20 minutes at 280 F. Serve up hot with bread.

Garlic Potatoes

Shopping List

- 4 Potatoes peeled and cut into cubes

- Olive oil

- Salt and pepper

- Marinated garlic

- Fresh rosemary

Instructions

Place a little oil and garlic in the Air Fryer at 360 F for 5 minutes. Half the time remove. Add the potatoes, the rosemary, salt, and pepper to taste and fry at 360 F for4 to 8 minutes. Half the time removes. Serve up as a chicken, meat or fish companion.

Buffalo's Tofu

Shopping List

- 400g tofu

- Cornstarch

- Olive oil

- 4 tablespoons of hot sauce

- ¼ cup of water

- Juice ½ lemon

- Soy sauce

- 40g cashew nuts

- Tarragon, thyme, dill, garlic powder, onion powder, paprika (1 teaspoon each)

- Pepper

Instructions

Reserve up 150g of tofu. Cut the rest into strips, and go through cornstarch. Place in the Air Fryer at 360 F for 8 to 12 minutes and allow cooling. In a bowl add the hot sauce and the same amount of oil. Mix and dip the fried tofu. Place in the Air Fryer programmed at 360 F for 15 to20 minutes. Meanwhile, add the rest of the Shopping Listto the blender and process until everything is integrated. Serve up the tofu with the sauce prepared.

Garbanzo's Tofu

Shopping List

- 1 cup chickpea flour

- 2 cups of water

- Salt

- Spices like curry or smoked paprika

- Olive oil

Instructions

Coat a preferential mold with oil. Mix all the Shopping List to taste in a pot, except the oil. Place on fire and stir vigorously. When the bubbles begin, reduce the heat and keep stirring for 3 minutes. Pour the mixture into the previously greased mold. Level the surface and let cool. Once at room temperature. Cover and Reserve up in the refrigerator overnight. Cut into cubes and add them to the Air Fryer, at 360 F for 5 15 minutes

Various Puff Pastry with Batter

Shopping List

- Various puff pastries

- Sliced eggplant

- Artichokes

- 1 sliced tomato

- Mayonnaise

- Salt

- 1 beaten egg

- Breadcrumbs

Instructions

Salt the eggplants and Reserve on absorbent paper for 10 minutes. Cut the artichokes in half and remove the fluff. Submerge in oil and cook over low heat until ten der. Drain and Reserve. Pass the eggplants and arti chokes for egg and bread. Polish everything with olive oil and add to the Air Fryer. Schedule at 300 F for 12 15 minutes. Serve up the puff pastry with the artichokes. Place tomato slices on the eggplants and a spoonful of mayonnaise on top.

Cassava Dumplings with Ciboulette

Shopping List

- 1½ kg of cassava

- 2 liters of water

- 1 teaspoon of salt

- 300 g of white cheese cut into cubes

- 12 sweet peppers cut into squares

- 4 cloves of garlic

- 1 pack of ciboulette cut into small pieces

- 1 cup of cut coriander leaves

- 1/2 cup olive oil

- Spicy to taste

- Salt and pepper

Instructions

Peel and cut the yucca. Place them to boil in salted water. When softening, crush them. Knead and form spheres by filling them with cheese. Accommodate the spheres in a tray and refrigerate. When they are soft, grind or grind them very well. Knead and make balls with cassava dough. Place a piece of cheese in the center of each bowl. Locate the balls in the mold of the Air Fryer. Freeze at 360 F for 8 to 12 minutes. Serve up with the sauce preferably.

Eggplant's Dice

Shopping List

- 1 Eggplant small cubes in water with salt

- ½ Onion in small cubes

- 1 grated tomato

- Salt

- 5 beaten eggs

Instructions

Add the onion to a sauté pan. Drain the eggplant and add it to the pan. Sauté over low heat. If there is much liquid remove it; add the tomato, salt, and stir. Add the mixture to the mold of the Air Fryer and add the eggs as well. Schedule at 340 F for 15 20 minutes. Serve up with bread and coffee.

Plantain's Tequeños

Shopping List

- 1 Ripe banana peeled

- ½ cup of wheat flour

- Olive oil

- 1 beaten egg

- Hard cheese cut into strips of 1 x 1 x 5cm

Instructions

Cook the banana in water. Add oil, salt, and puree. Add flour and knead until it has manageable dough. Place flour on the counter and stretch the dough with a rolling pin until it is thin. Cut strips of dough and varnish with egg. Place each strip of cheese and roll the dough over the cheese, sealing the edges. Place the small cheese pancake varnished with oil, in the mold of the Air Fryer previously varnished with oil, programmed at 360 F for 15 20 minutes. In the middle of cooking stir. Serve up with tomato sauce.

Crunchy Cheese Sticks

Shopping List

- Cheddar cheese in strips of 1.5 x 1.5 x 6 cm

- Manchego cheese in strips of 1.5 x 1.5 x 6 cm

- Paprika

- Garlic powder

- Pepper

- Salt

- Olive oil

- Breadcrumbs

- Egg

- Crushed corn flakes

Instructions

Freeze the cheese strips for one hour. Meanwhile, mix the bread with pepper, garlic, paprika, and Reserve up. Unite the egg with salt, pepper, garlic, paprika, beat, and Reserve up. Set aside the crushed corn flakes and set aside. Remove the cheese strips from the freezer. Pass them through the egg, Breadcrumbs, egg and finally the corn flakes. Place in the Air Fryer and set at 360 F for 5 to 10 minutes. Serve up with ketchup or any preferential sauce.

Pie Du Fro mage

Shopping List

- 1 pack of wafer's pies

- Grated mozzarella cheese

- 1 egg

- 50g parmesan

- Parsley finely cut

- Salt and pepper

- Olive oil

Instructions

Mix the mozzarella, parsley, parmesan, egg, salt, and pepper. Place a teaspoon of filling in the center of each of the wafers. Fold in half and seal with a fork. Place the varnished pies with oil in the Air Fryer programmed at 360 F for 5 8 minutes. Serve up hot.

Potatoes with Paprika

Shopping List

- 1Kg of potatoes

- 2 Red and green paprika

- Yeast wheat flour

- Water

- Salt

- Butter

- Olive oil

Instructions

Wash and peel the potatoes. Cut them into cubes and cook them in salted water for 10 15 minutes. Meanwhile, cut the peppers into julienne strips. Sauté the peppers with a pinch of salt. Reserve up. Make a mashed potato in hot adding butter to taste, and sauté. Add wheat flour and knead until smooth. Make discs with preferential size mass. Place them in the Air Fryer programmed at 360 F for 8 12 minutes. Serve up hot with preferential filling.

Breaded Eggs

Shopping List

- 8 eggs

- 2 butter spoons

- 60gr wheat flour

- ½L milk

- Nutmeg

- 100g cheese

- 1 beaten egg

- Breadcrumbs

- Olive oil

- Pepper

- Salt

Instructions

Cook the eggs in a pot with salt for 12 minutes. Remove them and submerge them in cold water. Peel and cut in half. Separate the yolks from the whites. Cut the cheese; Mix with the yolks and crush everything. In a saucepan melt the butter and add the flour. Mix until browning flour and remove from heat. Add half of the milk and mix with rods. Bring to a boil and add the rest of the milk, stirring constantly. Add a pinch of nutmeg, season to taste. Add the sausage mixture, mix and remove from heat. Allow cooling and fill in the whites giving rounded shapes.

Pass through egg and Breadcrumbs, varnish with olive oil and place in the Air Fryer programmed at 360 F for 5 8 minutes.

Serve up with salad.

Spheres Stuffed with Surprise Cream

Shopping List

- 500g wheat flour

- 100g sugar

- Salt

- 4 eggs

- 150ml water

- 15g baking powder

- Grated ½ lemon

- 125g butter ointment

- Olive oil

- Preferential cream

Instructions

Add the yeast and 70g of sugar in the water, dilute and steep for 5 minutes. In the mixer add flour, salt, eggs, lemon zest and the water with yeast. Process until a homogeneous mixture is obtained. Place the butter little by little without stopping the mixer. When fully integrated, count 10 minutes and stop the mixer. Place in a bowl varnished with oil and cover with plastic wrap. Let stand for 1 hour. Knead by hand sprinkling little flour. Let rest again until the dough has twice its size. Cut pieces of ap proximately 45g and form balls. Place on individual pieces of butter paper, cover with a cloth and let stand for 2 hours.

Place inside the Air Fryer programmed at 360 F for 15 25 minutes. Half cooked cover with aluminum foil.

Sprinkle with sugar. Fill with preferential cream and a sleeve with the mouthpiece.

Serve up with tea or coffee.

Spinach Cocotets

Shopping List

- 1 pack of wafers for dumplings

- 300g defrosted and drained spinach

- 1 onion in julienne

- 3 garlic, mashed

- Olive oil

- White cheese in cubes

- Salt

Instructions

Sauté the onions with the garlic. When obtaining color add the spinach, salt and sauté for 5 minutes. Place the filling in the center of the wafers and some cheese. Rinse the edges with water and close by lifting the edges forming a drop. Coat with olive oil and place in the Air Fryer programmed at 360 F for 5 10 minutes. Serve up hot

Camembert with Strawberry Jam

Shopping List

- 300g Camembert at room temperature

- Wheat flour

- Breadcrumbs

- 2 beaten eggs

- Pepper and oregano to taste

- Olive oil

- Strawberry jam

Instructions

Cut the cheese and pass it through flour, egg, and bread. Place it in the Air Fryer programmed at 360 F for 3 6 minutes. Serve up sprinkling marmalade on top.

Spinach Lollipops

Shopping List

- Béchamel thick

- 2 tablespoons of flour

- 1 onion

- 1 cup of cooked rice

- Salt and pepper

- 300g of spinach leaves

- Olive oil

Instructions

Pass the spinach through boiling water for 1 minute. Process the onion, spinach, rice and salt and pepper. Take out the dough and knead with 2 tablespoons of flour. Form the croquettes and bathe with the béchamel sauce. Place in the refrigerator for 30 minutes. Take the Air Fryer programmed at 360 F for 8 12 minutes. Pierce with chopsticks and Serve up with cream cheese.

Pisto with Coffee

Shopping List

- 1 onion, 1 leek, 2 green and red peppers, 1 zucchini (julienne)

- 400g chopped tomato

- Olive oil

- Salt and pepper, and sugar

- 1 cup of coffee

- 6 tablespoons fried tomato

Instructions

In the mold of the Air Fryer add onions, leeks, peppers, zucchini and a little oil, mix and sauté at 400 F for 15 minutes. Remove periodically. Add the tomato, season and cook for 20 minutes. Remove periodically. After 5 minutes, add the fried tomato, coffee, and sugar to taste. Stir. Serve up with rice.

Pasties with Blanket

Shopping List

- 1 package of dough for dumplings

- Milk

- Butter

- Wheat flour

- Salt

- 1 beaten egg

- Breadcrumbs

- Olive oil

Instructions

Heat the milk with the butter until melted. Integrate wheat flour and salt to taste and mix until thick. Lower the heat and let it rest. Cool in fridge. Fill the masses and seal. Submerge them in the mixture and drain the excess. Place in the mold of the Air Fryer, varnished with oil and programmed at 360 F for 5 10 minutes. Serve up alone and accompany it by coffee or juice.

Vegetable Spaghetti

Shopping List

- 2 Washed courgettes

- 200g cottage cheese

- 100g sprouted

- 5 kinds of garlic, mashed

- Parsley finely cut

- Basil finely cut

- Parmesan

- The juice of 1 lime

- Salt and pepper

- Olive oil

Instructions

Cut the ends of the zucchini and cut into slices. Cut into thin strips to make the spaghetti. Sauté the garlic, add color to the zucchini and sauté. Add the herbs and incorporate them well. Add the cottage cheese, parmesan and salt, and pepper. Skip well to integrate everything. Spray the lime juice and add the sprouts. Sauté 1 minute and remove from heat. Serve up hot

Homemade Guacamole

Shopping List

- 8 corn tortillas

- Olive oil

- 2 Avocados

- 1 Tomato, 1 Onion and ½ Chives (finely chopped)

- Finely sliced coriander

- Juice of 1 Lima

- Salt

Instructions

Cut the tortillas in 4.

Place in the Air Fryer at 360 F for 3 – 5 minutes.

Remove the meat from the avocados and mash.

Add the onion, green onion and tomato and mix.

Add the coriander, salt and mix well. Add lime juice and mix.

Serve up the fake nachos with the guacamole.

French Donuts

Shopping List

- 7g yeast dissolved in 175ml water

- 115ml evaporated milk

- 1 egg

- 50g sugar

- ½ teaspoon of salt

- 440g wheat flour

- 25g ointment butter

- Olive oil

- Sugar glass

Instructions

In a bowl, mix milk, egg, sugar, and salt. Incorporate the yeast, and add the flour little by little. When it is well beaten, add the butter. In the inn, flour and place the dough. Knead until smooth. Cover with film and Reserve up in the fridge for 24 hours. Flour the counter, knead and stretch with the help of a rolling pin, until it is 1cm thick. Shape with a cutter, varnish with olive oil. Take the Air Fryer programmed at 360 F for 8 15 minutes. Sprinkle icing sugar and Serve up with coffee or chocolate.

Puffers Fritter

Shopping List

- 400g Pumpkin without skin

- 450g Wheat flour

- 125ml Cooking water

- Sugar

- 7g Salt

- 25g Fresh Yeast

- Orange zest

- Olive oil

Instructions

Cut the squash into large cubes and boil in plenty of water for 20 minutes. Take out and Reserve. Dissolve the yeast in 125ml of cooking water. Crush the pumpkin to obtain a paste. Mix the pumpkin, yeast, 20g of sugar, or ange zest and 7g of salt. Add the sifted flour a little and stir until everything is integrated. Let stand for 15 minutes covered with plastic wrap. Wet your hands in oil and form the fritters with a hole in the center and place in the Air Fryer varnished with olive oil, programmed at 360 F for 8 12 minutes. Sprinkle with sugar and Serve up with coffee.

French Toast's Stuffed with Milk Candy

Shopping List

- 1 breadstick

- 1liter milk

- Tangerine grated

- Lemon zest

- Caramel

- 5 tablespoons sugar

- 3 eggs

- Vanilla

- 1 cinnamon branch

- Mixed sugar and cinnamon

Instructions

In a pot, boil the milk, the tangerine and lemon zest, cinnamon, vanilla, and sugar. Beat the eggs, cut the bread into slices of 1 centimeter. Bathe the bread in the milk, put two together. Fill with milk candy. Pass them through the beaten egg and bring to the mold of the Air Fryer painted with oil. Program it at 360 F for 5 10 minutes. Sprinkle with sugar and cinnamon. Serve up with coffee, tea or hot milk.

Nachos with Yogurt

Shopping List

- 1 Package Corn Tortillas

- Olive oil

- A natural yogurt

- ½ lemon juice

- Parsley cut

- Salt and pepper

Instructions

Cut the corn tortillas into 8 triangles. Bathe with olive oil and place in the Air Fryer programmed at 360 F for 5 10 minutes. While in the blender, add yogurt, a little oil, lemon juice, parsley and salt and pepper to taste. Processes until obtaining the desired thickness. Serve up the nachos with the yogurt sauce.

Poached Potatoes

Shopping List

- Olive oil.

- Sliced potatoes

- 1 julienne onion

- 2 red and green chili peppers julienne

- 2 kinds of garlic, mashed

- Salt

- Oregano.

- Parsley finely cut.

- Minced garlic

- Vinegar

Instructions

In the mold of the Air Fryer, heat a little oil at 360 F for 5 minutes. Add the onions, potatoes, peppers, garlic, and salt. Stir and program it at 360 F for 20 minutes. Mix periodically. Missing 5 minutes, add oregano, parsley, vinegar, ground. Remove and finish the programming. Serve up hot as a garnish.

Nachos with Cheese

Shopping List

- 300g Wheat flour

- 3 teaspoons of salt

- 1 teaspoon hot pepper powder

- 2 teaspoons garlic powder

- 1 teaspoon curry

- ½ teaspoon cumin powder

- ½ teaspoon ground cayenne

- 1 pinch of sugar

- 10g fresh yeast

- 150ml water

- Olive oil and 1 glass of sunflower oil

- Grated cheddar cheese

- Grated mozzarella cheese

Instructions

Mix salt, hot paprika, garlic, curry, cumin, cayenne, and sugar. In the mixer dissolve yeast in the water. Add flour, 20g of the previous mixture, oil and knead until smooth. Make balls of approximately 50g. Stretch with a roller until you get discs. Cook in a skillet over medium high heat for 1 minute. Flip, cook 15 seconds and re move. Cut 3 times in half and varnish with olive oil. Place the triangles in the Air Fryer, programming at 300 F for 8 15 minutes.

In the mold of the Air Fryer alternate layers of nachos and cheese.

If you want, boost the spice by placing chilies. Schedule at 360 F for 12 15 minutes.

Serve up with some extra nachos on top.

Sweet Tortillas

Shopping List

- 1 package of wheat tortillas

- 50g sugar

- Cinnamon powder

- Olive oil

Instructions

Mix the cinnamon and sugar. Coat the tortillas with olive oil and place them in the Air Fryer. Program it at 360 F for 3 8 minutes. If necessary, half cooked, turn. Sprinkle with a colander the sugar mixture. Serve up and taste hot or cold with coffee or juice.

CONCLUSION

The new cooking system that Air Fryer has was designed especially thinking about how to prepare food with a reduction of fat by 75%, which translates into health benefits. The Instructionsof food with a minimum amount of oil, requires the cooking process with the natural fats of food, resulting in a healthy diet, which contributes to the reduction of the problem of overweight, and at the same time prevents the appearance of diseases of modern life, produced by excess fat in the body due to poor diet.

Air Fryer arrived to provide a better quality of life option for all people who wish to improve their diet and enjoy a full life with their loved ones.

In the present eBook, you have more than 1000 options to prepare your food in a free and fun way, to make combinations to your liking and of your loved ones, with a minimum of oil, in its natural and crispy fats on the outside and juices inside. Remember, the processes of preparing recipes may vary if you have knowledge in cooking. If the proportions of the Shopping Listprovided are respected, you will find the best flavors for your recipes, and your journey into using an air fryer will drastically cut down on the unhealthy, fried foods.

With the air fryer, you will discover a different flavor, but it's very similar to what you already know. The only real difference the air fryer makes is the amount of fat in your food. Invest in an air fryer and take the time to prolong your life by becoming a healthier version of yourself

Try them!

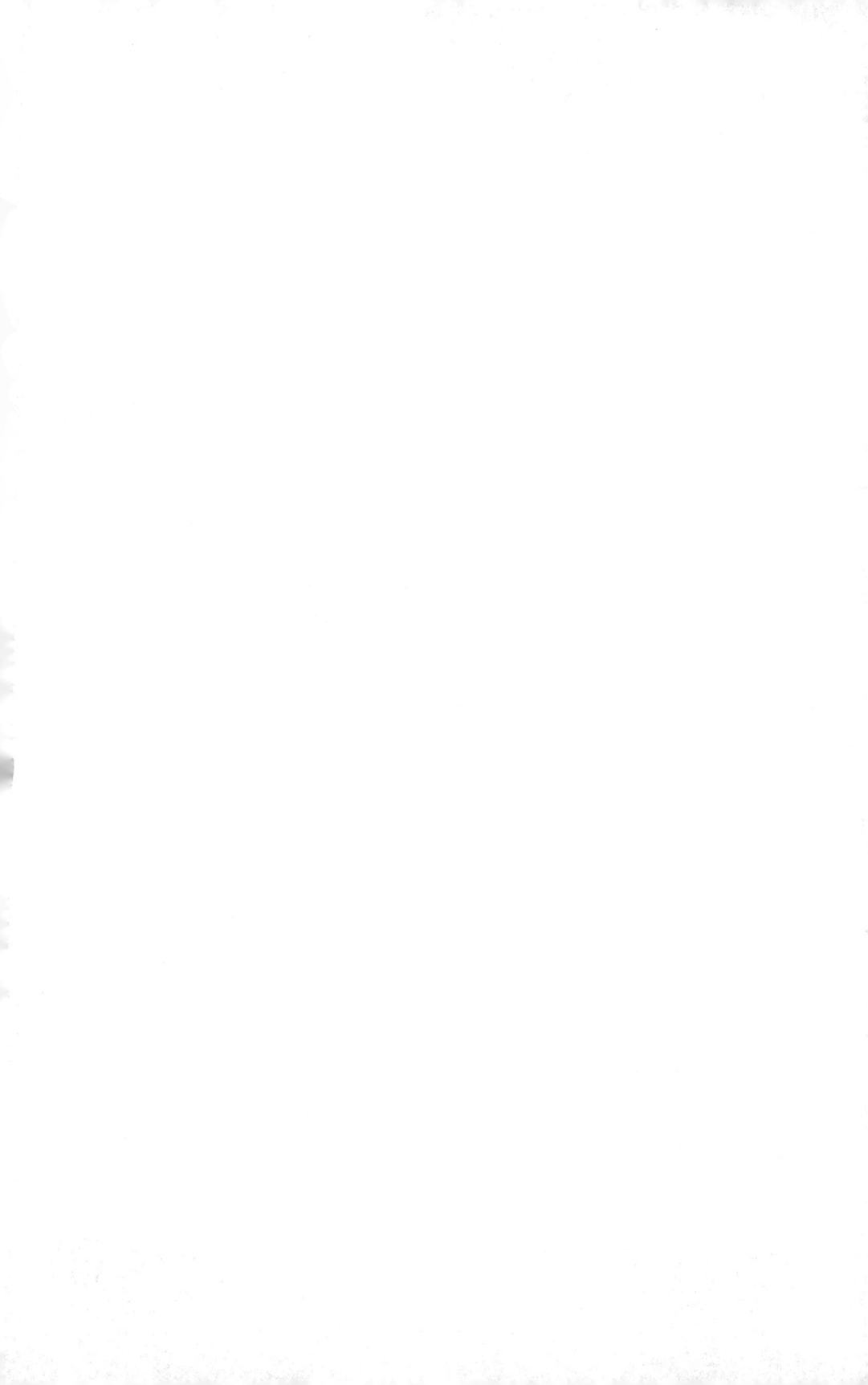

CPSIA information can be obtained
at www.ICGtesting.com
Printed in the USA
BVHW042132080621
609011BV00012B/2569

9 781802 572001